I0707108

My Journey Through Congestive Heart Failure

by E. Gordon Mooneyhan

My Journey Through Congestive Heart Failure

Copyright 2020 by E. Gordon Mooneyhan

ISBN: 9798648679344

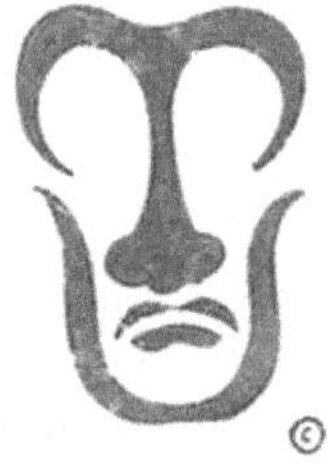

Sea Island Publishing

P.O. Box 2328

Myrtle Beach, SC 29578

Other Books by E. Gordon Mooneyhan

The Atlantic Coast Line Railroad Dining Car Cookbook

The Seaboard Air Line Railroad Dining Car Cookbook

The Southern Railway Dining Car Cookbook

Public Relations for the Volunteer Public Information Officer

VI

DEDICATION

There are so many people to thank because, without their help and guidance, I wouldn't be here today. I dedicate this book to all the doctors and nurses who made it possible for me to be here today. Thanks to all of you for not only saving my life but also for giving me the opportunity to have a new outlook for the rest of my life.

This isn't intended to be a medical book by any stretch of the imagination, and I'm sure that I've confused some of the tests and what they were designed to do. I wasn't thinking about writing a book when I was diagnosed. If I had, I would have kept better notes. In fact, the idea for this book didn't really occur until after the surgery. Rather, this is the book I wish I had access to when I was first diagnosed with congestive heart failure and when I was told that my Mitral Valve would need to be repaired. That is a book telling me what to expect as I traveled along this voyage of discovery, and of self-discovery. Nothing is worse than not knowing, or if you prefer the more traditional saying, knowledge is power.

Last but certainly not least, I am indebted to Sunny Fry and Janet Reitzel for taking the time to proofread the first draft and suggest needed edits. Any typos are my responsibility.

"The art of medicine consists in amusing the patient while nature cures the disease." Voltaire

"A hospital bed is a parked taxi with the meter running." Groucho Marx

CONTENTS

On April 1, 2019, I was diagnosed with congestive heart failure. About a month earlier, I had made a large food delivery to a baseball field complex in Myrtle Beach, SC. I started to lose my breath while shuffling the food between my car and the customer. I got back in my car and sat, with the air conditioning running, for about 10 minutes. Although I hadn't fully caught my breath, I did feel well enough to drive back to work, and that was my last delivery of the day. I was off from work for the next two days and took it easy, spending the time resting.

I still wasn't feeling 100%. I made the decision that if I wasn't feeling better in a week to 10 days, that I would go to a doctor. You know how things go when you put them off—you forget about time. Long story short, I ended up going to the doctor on April 1st, April Fool's Day.

The diagnosis was less than appealing. When I was told I had congestive heart failure, my first reply was, "That's not a good April Fool's joke." Once I was assured it was no joke, the reality set in of how long do I have left? As far as I knew, congestive heart failure was a death sentence; not an immediate death sentence, but three to five years.

Like most people, I don't keep up with medical advances that's something that, at the time, was not in my zone of awareness. I did know that heart disease was the leading cause of death in the United States. My doctor was quick to set me straight. Congestive heart failure was no longer a death sentence. Although there is no cure, with proper diet, exercise, and medication, it would be manageable and I could expect to have a relatively "normal" life expectancy.

That news gave me an entirely new mindset, one where I realized that I could have a great rest of my life. That mental change, in turn, led to me researching what was healthy, what wasn't, what might be good for me, etc.

What follows in this book are my thoughts on diet, exercise, maintaining one's health, etc. Let me start with this disclaimer: I AM NOT A DOCTOR. Before making any changes to your health regimen, talk it over with your doctor first. Also, I am making a concerted effort to avoid or minimize medical jargon. This isn't intended to be a textbook, but rather a layperson's book to help give an idea of what to expect. Nothing is worse than not knowing. Also, it's quite likely, that I have confused some of the tests and what they were supposed to do. Again, this isn't a medical textbook rather it is a record of what I experienced, and I share it to give you knowledge. It's information that I wish I had known before my journey started, which would have made the voyage less stressful.

What I will do in these pages is share with you the changes I made in my life. I invite you to come along on my journey, share and hopefully learn from my mistakes. Along the way, I'll also share doctor's visits, learning about congestive heart failure, and some other medical information.

Lastly, remember that YOU ARE YOUR OWN BEST ADVOCATE FOR YOUR CARE! Yes, I meant to "shout" that, because it needed to be shouted.

"You know, if I listened to Michael Dukakis long enough, I would be convinced we're in an economic downturn and people are homeless and going without food and medical attention and that we've got to do something about the unemployed." Ronald Reagan

"Getting out of the hospital is a lot like resigning from a book club. You're not out of it until the computer says you're out of it." Erma Bombeck

CHAPTER ONE THE DIAGNOSIS

Getting diagnosed with any life-threatening disease is, for most people, a wake-up call. It's a sign from the Almighty that you need to, as the old song said, "Straighten up and fly right." However, there are those who will, in spite of what doctors say, continue down their reckless path.

A prime example is the following. My dad had a triple bypass. After the surgery he and one other person locally were signed up for an experimental heart treatment called Dobutamine. They were both told that, if they followed the doctor's instructions, they could expect about an additional five years of relatively normal life. Dad followed the doctor's instructions pretty much to the letter. The other person really loved bowling and continued to bowl even though it was against the doctor's advice. The other person died after only about 2½ years. Dad got a few months over five years and was in remarkably good health until just about a month before he died. My point is that, even though you are your own best advocate for your health, listen to the doctor. S/he will know best.

Speaking of listening, learn to listen to your body. Congestive heart failure is insidious; it creeps up on you slowly. The symptoms, such as shortness of breath, creep up. Your body starts to retain water, again slowly. Your weight slowly increases. It may eventually stabilize at some point as mine did. I'm five feet, eight inches tall. My weight crept up from 190 to 225 pounds and then held there. It was a slow weight gain, nothing that would be alarming. All the symptoms were slow to come, so slow that most people would just see them as a sign of growing older, not as an alarm that anything was wrong. It was that way with me. I just assumed that it was a collection of signs that I had reached 62 and I would have to start slowing down.

As I said in the introduction, I went to the doctor on April 1st and received the diagnosis. After the shock and the wisecrack reply about it being a bad April Fool's joke and then being told it wasn't a joke, but it also wasn't the end of my life either, I realized that yes, this could be a new beginning, a new chance to get to experience life. Upon reflection, this was the sunset of my old life.

Once I got the diagnosis, I realized that my ankles were very swollen. When I was about six months old, I was in the hospital for about two months, having premature closure of the scalp. There is a scar on my left ankle that looks kind of like a tic tac toe board. It's where the IV tubes were connected. My ankles were so swollen that the skin had stretched to the point that I couldn't see or feel that scar anymore. This is one of the things I mean about listening to your body.

The congestive heart failure diagnosis came with a host of medicines, especially Lasix. Lasix makes your body shed excess water by urination. It's a case of you don't want to get too far away from a bathroom. The first week, I was going about every 20 to 30 minutes. That was fun, especially when I was trying to deliver food. I remember getting to one office, making the delivery, and asking if I could borrow their restroom because I knew I wouldn't be able to make it back to work. Yes, there are big life changes like that. There were other medicines, mainly to control my blood pressure, and the effects of those are easy to feel (lightheadedness being the major side effect). There was one point where I was taking seven or eight prescriptions each day. Some were once a day, some twice daily, and there was one that was three times each day.

Although it seems counterintuitive, if you are retaining fluids and on Lasix, you need to drink plenty of water. I know, your objective is to lose excess water so why would you want to drink more? When you are thirsty, your body's natural reaction is to reduce fluid loss, which is to retain fluids. Since you want to lose fluids, you must drink more. Plain and simple.

There are also smaller life changes. Pizza went from being a weekly treat to maybe one or two slices a month. Tomato sauce is high in sodium (salt) and sodium makes you retain water.

Although I was born in Connecticut, I was raised in the south. I learned to love southern food—fried chicken, sweet iced tea, homemade biscuits, you get the idea. Surprisingly, fried chicken was relatively easy to handle. I still enjoy it, but now I don't eat the skin. I know, the skin is where the flavor is, but that flavor includes salt. I know there are salt substitutes, but those are, in my opinion, fraught with their own health hazards. Sweet iced tea has been my Achilles Heel. I loved it to the point that I was drinking it morning, noon, and night, about a gallon a day. I won't use any artificial sweeteners as I can't get used to the aftertaste, so now I just cut way back to one or two glasses a week. And if I go to a place where I can serve myself, I'll do about ¼ sweet and ¾ unsweet. I'll talk more about food adjustments later when I get to lifestyle changes—I refuse to use the word diet.

There were a lot of changes that I had to make. I didn't make them suddenly, but rather I paced myself in making the changes. It's like driving a car on a slick road in the rain. If you turn too hard, the car will skid out of control. Gradual turns will keep you on the road. In the same way, I did my lifestyle changes, slow but sure, making sure I would stay on the road and not go skidding off.

"It is in moments of illness that we are compelled to recognize that we live not alone but chained to a creature of a different kingdom, whole worlds apart, who has no knowledge of us and by whom it is impossible to make ourselves understood: our body." Marcel Proust

"If my doctor told me I only had six minutes to live, I wouldn't brood. I'd type a little faster." Isaac Asimov

CHAPTER TWO MORE BAD NEWS

I was doing fine losing weight, averaging between one and two pounds each day. I had to keep a log for the doctor of my weight each morning and blood pressure both morning and evening (I still keep it). I ended up making an Excel spreadsheet to track those figures, and it made it easy to just print out a copy when I needed to see the doctor. Also, since not even the CIA can decipher my handwriting, having it neatly typed was the best option and assured no mistakes on my part.

Even though the weight was dropping off, I wasn't regaining my breath. My General Practitioner was somewhat concerned and she made an appointment for me to visit a lab for an Electrocardiogram (EKG), just to get a better picture of what was going on with my heart.

I showed up at the appointed time and had about a half dozen electrodes attached to me. About an hour of poking and prodding followed, including time with an ultrasonic wand to get a better idea of what was happening. The lab results were sent to a cardiologist and eventually back to my doctor when I got the call to come in to talk about what they had discovered.

I had a leaking heart valve and I would have to go down to Tidelands Hospital in Georgetown for tests. The appointed day arrives and I get a ride down to the hospital. I get checked in, then it's a game of "hurry up and wait." Eventually, I'm brought into the room where they will run a catheter through my veins to see how things are. They initially go in through my groin. I only have bits and pieces of a recollection here. I do remember being awake for part of the procedure and watching the probe on a TV monitor as it was moved around in my heart. I do remember not feeling anything from it. Eventually, they go through my wrist to finish the test. Their (incorrect) conclusion, was that I had some major blockage in my Aorta, the main artery where blood leaves the heart and gets sent to the rest of your body.

This procedure was supposed to be outpatient, meaning that I would be going home the same day. It ended up being an overnight stay because it was so late when the procedure ended Also there was a lack of communication and I ended up being put in a regular room instead of a recovery room. Not having a change of clothes or toiletries made for a very unpleasant night at the hospital. I wish I had been told of the possibility that I would need to spend the night. At least having toiletries would have made it less stressful.

My ride home from the hospital was uneventful, although I was, along with my friend who picked me up, amazed at the lack of communication among the hospital staff. It was almost as if some of them didn't know what was going on, and it was my opinion that they were thrown in to take care of me with no knowledge of my condition. Yes, I can get cynical.

The net result of this was the conclusion that I should get a second opinion to look at the issues. Fortunately for me, that would require more tests, this time at the Medical University of South Carolina (MUSC), in Charleston. And it was indeed fortunate, as the tests would reveal the incorrect diagnosis made at Tidelands Hospital.

I think it's important to state at this point that I don't consider what happened at Tidelands to be malpractice. No surgery or medication was affected because of the misdiagnosis. Nothing that potentially threatened my life occurred because of the misdiagnosis.

"As a surgeon, you have to have a controlled arrogance. If it's uncontrolled, you kill people, but you have to be pretty arrogant to saw through a person's chest, take out their heart and believe you can fix it. Then, when you succeed and the patient survives, you pray, because it's only by the grace of God that you get there." Mehmet Oz

"Keep a watch also on the faults of the patients, which often make them lie about taking the things prescribed." Hippocrates

CHAPTER THREE THE WAITING GAME

Waiting is the worst part. I had a couple of visits with a cardiologist from Tidelands for prescriptions to regulate my blood pressure. At the same time, I was forced to cut back on the amount of work I was doing. Food delivery is strenuous exercise. Granted, it's not continuous, but it does require a certain amount of energy; a high output over short spans of time.

It got to the point that I was having to use a cane when I would walk to some of the hotel rooms in the area, simply because of the distance involved. During this time, my weight had dropped from a high of 225 pounds down to 160 pounds. I was feeling wonderful, mentally. I was having to wear a belt again, and I could tuck my shirt in. When I weighed 225 pounds, I wore my shirts untucked whenever possible because I was embarrassed by the way I looked—like I was two months past due and pregnant with twins. It eventually reached the point that I couldn't deliver food anymore, because it was just too exhausting to try to carry food to the rooms or homes. Mentally I was fine, but physically I was a wreck.

During all of this, my employer was wonderful. South Carolina is a right to work state, meaning you can be terminated without cause. Technically, I could have been fired. Instead, they initially asked me to work four or five evenings a week, sitting on my tush and answering the phones—a glorified order taker. Eventually, I was cut back to three times a week, and then, after the surgery, I was told to come in when I wanted. Inevitably I would be sent home after an hour or two because they had to watch the labor costs. More on that later.

I don't know which is worse, waiting, or not knowing exactly what is wrong. Both cause mental strain on you, but they are different types of strain, or maybe different sides of the same strain. Waiting is hard because you don't know what the course of action will be. In many ways, not knowing what is wrong causes the same type of strain. You don't know so your mind starts running through options. You try hard not to go down that path because you end up dealing with false hopes.

At this point, I still did not know that I had been misdiagnosed by Tidelands Health, and I wouldn't know that until I would meet with my cardiologist at MUSC. I had several months of waiting, not knowing, thinking there was something wrong that really wasn't wrong. And all this time the anxiety kept building.

About this time, I started doing online research, trying to learn about my condition, what options there were for surgery and, most important, was there anything I could do to be proactive in my care. I know enough to be skeptical about what I may see on the Internet. At the same time, knowledge is power. Knowledge also helped take my mind off the uncertainty that I was facing. I think that's an important point when one is facing the unknown you need to replace the unknown with a known. Even if it turns out later that the knowledge is wrong, having a solid point of focus gives peace of mind.

"We can't let people down when they can't get any medical care when they're sick and don't have money to go to a doctor. You help them." Donald Trump

"Disease is an experience of a so-called mortal mind. It is fear made manifest on the body." Mary Baker Eddy

CHAPTER FOUR CHANGES TO MY LIFESTYLE

The biggest single change in my life was lifestyle changes. Eating was a big part of the change but I refuse to use the word "diet" because diet implies sacrifice, and there is much more to lifestyle changes than food.

I started making these changes before I had the first meeting with my cardiologist down at MUSC. There were three major points to my lifestyle change plan, a trident if you will.

The first, and probably the biggest change, was in my mindset. A positive mental attitude works wonders. You start facing the world with an attitude of "I can" instead of "I can't." Trust me, it makes a difference, and that positive attitude changes your entire outlook on the rest of your life. It makes the remaining changes much, much easier.

There are proponents of having a positive mental attitude who suggest that you make a list of your positive attributes. I didn't do that. Rather, I focused on a mindset that the surgery would be successful and I would be in better health after it was over. Did that help? Who knows? I remember being told on the Monday of surgery that I would probably be released the following Saturday. I remember waking up in the ICU at about 3 AM on Tuesday when they were taking my vital signs. My cardiologist, Doctor Katz, came by later in the morning and told me the surgery had gone well and that I would likely be released on Saturday. He came by on Thursday and said, "We're releasing you today." Did my mental attitude have anything to do with that? I don't know, but I choose to believe that it did, and no one can convince me otherwise.

Food choices were the second biggest factor for me. I love to eat and I love trying new recipes. I'll admit it, I'm a Food Network junkie. Living alone, I used to spend a good portion of time in grocery stores going through the canned goods. The problem with canned food is that it has a fairly high salt (sodium) content. My doctor told me that fact when I was diagnosed. She strongly suggested that I should find a diet plan that

I could live with, and Lord knows, the bookstores are filled with cookbooks advocating the virtues of various diets.

As I've said, I dislike the word "diet" because of the connotations it creates in one's mind. I began perusing the various cookbooks in my favorite bookstore. I looked at Atkins, Keto, and various other diets ad nauseum. I'm not knocking any of these diets. If you find one that works for you, that's great. I eventually settled on a "Modified" Mediterranean Diet. I liked the philosophy of fresh food. That got me away from the canned goods. It also got me to start eating fresh fruits for snacks, oranges and bananas being my favorites. I also settled on chicken as a primary protein. I know what you must be thinking, "Gordon, how can you eat chicken all the time?" I said primary protein, not sole protein. Chicken is very versatile. It accepts marinades fairly well, so the flavor and texture of the meat can vary. I do visit the canned food aisle in grocery stores for tuna (in water, not oil). A couple of times a week I'll enjoy a tuna salad, using a combination of mayonnaise and mustard to add flavor to the salad.

Another side of my "Modified" Mediterranean Diet is the wok. I know, a wok is primarily used for Chinese food, but I "adapt" some of the recipes. Olive oil for the oil, stir-fry the veggies with maybe just a touch of light soy sauce.

I once had a chef tell me that cooking and baking were like art and science. Cooking is an art; the recipe is a basic guide that you can tweak for your own personal taste. Baking is more like science. It's much harder to adjust the recipe to achieve the same result.

As anyone who has heart problems knows, sodium (salt) is something to avoid. It increases blood pressure, makes the body retain fluids, and in general isn't all that healthy for you. But at the same time, it is an easy way to add flavor which is why most prepared foods contain sodium, and if you look at the amount, you'll see that it's pretty much all you need. The prepackaged frozen dinners are the same way. Fortunately, I didn't make a habit of those meals, maybe only two or three times a year. Now, I just avoid them, period.

In one of Mel Brooks' "2000-Year-Old Man" recordings, he says, "We mock the thing we are to be." I remember being younger and going grocery shopping and, quietly to myself, mock the older shoppers who were looking at the nutrition information on each label. Guess what, that's me now. We mock the thing we are to be. Yep, I'm reading the nutrition labels now.

I also love nuts, cashews in particular. I tried eating unsalted, using a homemade dry ranch seasoning, but I wasn't crazy about it. I ended up buying lightly salted cashews since they have less than half the salt of regular cashews. Also, while too much sodium is bad, the body needs some to be able to function. I compromise with the lightly salted cashews and, when I buy them, I make sure to buy less of other salted items, in other words, I look at the sodium content a bit closer than usual.

Speaking of avoiding other salted items, processed meats (salami, pepperoni, ham, etc.) are all high in sodium and I have, for the most part, crossed them off my shopping list.

While I was in the hospital, as a routine part of the check, my blood sugar was checked and I was diagnosed as borderline diabetic. Now I not only check sodium, but I also check for sugar. It wasn't that hard to cut sugar; I was already doing that as part of my lifestyle change. As I said, sweet iced tea has been cut back to one or two times a week. My first blood sugar check was on Tuesday and, by Thursday, I was no longer borderline diabetic. So now I watch the carbohydrates in addition to sodium. It's all part of the total equation of life.

I think the best possible course of action is to follow Julia Child's advice—moderation. I admit that I'm not a great physical specimen, but I see customers come into work to order food and they have to, for lack of a better term, waddle. Three, maybe four hundred pounds. The road that I've been on has made me more aware of others. And no, I don't say anything derogatory to them. Fat-shaming someone won't do any good. They have to want to make the change for themselves. No one can do it for them. And no one can do it for you.

The last prong of my lifestyle change trident is exercise. And it has been the hardest for me to do. I can't exercise for the sake of exercising. A gym doesn't work for me. I can't tell you how much money I wasted on gym memberships over my life. I'd join, go maybe three times, and forget about it. I did start mall walking. Before the surgery, I was averaging about ¼ mile each day. As I write this, I'm 30 days post-surgery and I'm up to about ½ mile each day, with an occasional one-mile day thrown in for good measure. I'm also back at work delivering food about three days a week. I average close to a mile of walking on those days, although it's in short spurts, not one long stretch. But that really doesn't solve the exercise problem for me. I have a road bike at home, an older Schwinn, and I'll start getting back on it once the warmer weather starts, and once I've been cleared for exercise. As of now, cardiac rehab was scheduled to begin in February but has been postponed to May because of Covid-19.

We make changes to our lifestyles after something has been diagnosed, and the changes are to correct what we've managed to foul up. A prime example for me is starting an exercise routine instead of having done it since day one to prevent the problems from occurring in the first place. If you take away nothing else, take this. The changes are like preventive maintenance on a car. Take care of yourself now so you'll have a longer, healthier life later.

"If a person is treated like a patient, they are apt to act like one." Frances Farmer

"My doctor gave me six months to live, but when I couldn't pay the bill, he gave me six months more." Walter Matthau

CHAPTER FIVE PREPARING FOR SURGERY

Prior to my surgery, I had to make about a half dozen trips down to MUSC for diagnosis and tests in preparation for the surgery. The first one I had a friend drive me, simply because I didn't want to face the potential bad news alone. All of my tests and surgery took place at the MUSC Ashley River Tower.

It's hard to remember exactly what happened when, but I'll give it my best shot. At the time, the thought of writing a book hadn't entered my mind, so I really didn't keep notes.

The first trip to MUSC included an EKG, a CAT scan, and a heart catheterization, as well as a meeting with two cardiologists, one of whom, Dr. Marc Katz, would eventually perform the surgery on me.

The heart catheterization was probably the most informative test of the lot. That was the test that showed Tidelands Hospital had made a mistake. They had forced the catheter into the wall of one of my veins and read it as a blockage instead of the wall of the vein.

In meeting with the doctors, I was given the bad news. The damage could be repaired, but it would have to be open heart surgery which would require between eight and twelve weeks of recovery. I thought, well at least there is hope, there is a solution to the problem.

An appointment was then made for a couple of weeks later for some additional tests, the worst of which was a trans-esophageal EKG. This would require a tranquilizer and a tube that would be inserted down my esophagus. With that, they would be able to get more accurate pressure readings and have a better idea of what was going on with my heart, as the esophagus would allow the sensor to be very close to my heart, as opposed to having to get a reading from outside the body. This would allow for much more accurate readings. I was told that I would need someone to drive me home because I was going to be sedated. This would prove to be a problem because I really didn't want to impose on someone to drive me down, spend an entire day at the hospital (other tests were also going to be performed), and then have to drive me home.

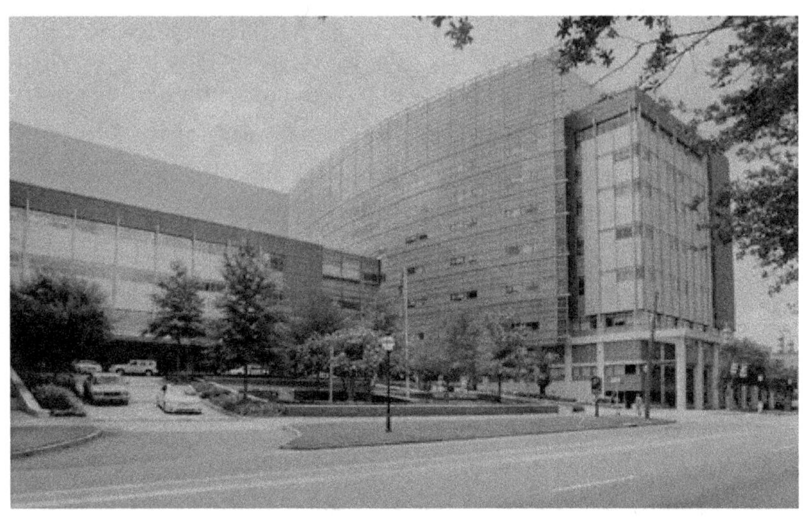

MUSC Ashley River Tower, where all my doctor visits and surgery occurred.

I do some freelance business consulting. I was able to line a job up for the day after this procedure in Charleston, and I found a hotel that would let me leave my car in their lot while I was at the hospital. I would then spend the night at the hotel (the Holiday Inn at the Ashley River), and the next day I would do my job and drive home.

Before being sedated, I had to gargle with a solution to numb my throat, and it had to be the worst tasting stuff imaginable. Other than the God-awful taste, I really don't remember much of anything from that test. How bad did it taste? I still gag thinking about it.

There was also a CAT scan that day. It was mostly painless.

There was a third trip down for more tests. I have to admit that I was getting frustrated with the tests. The best analogy would be a picture versus a movie. A picture is a snapshot, a single moment. A movie helps to present the whole picture. You get a view that tells the whole story, or as much of the story as can be told before seeing firsthand with the surgery. That's what the tests were doing, they were helping to provide a complete picture of my heart. I realized this after the fact, but it would have been nice if it had been explained ahead of time.

At the same time, the news was getting better after each series of tests. After the second set of tests, it was thought that they could do the surgery by going in through one of my veins. That is less invasive which means much quicker recovery time. After the third series of tests, it was determined that I was a prime candidate for robotic surgery. There would be five incisions made at my ribs, along with a couple of drains. I can remember watching Star Trek as a kid, and Doctor McCoy was standing over the patient, with a "box" over the patient's chest. McCoy was twisting dials on the box, performing surgery. Yeah, right, that will never happen. Well, it has happened. My doctor repaired my mitral valve using a DaVinci robot to help him perform the surgery.

They say you can find anything on the Internet. It's true. I found a condensed video of the mitral valve surgery (about 15 minutes in length). I also found a video of the DaVinci robot being used by a doctor to peel a grape.

YouTube video of the DaVinci Robot peeling a grape:

https://www.youtube.com/watch?v=cpPofyZbvDw

While I was getting the good news, I still had feelings of uncertainty. This leads to the next chapter about second opinions.

"Thinking of disease constantly will intensify it. Feel always 'I am healthily in body and mind." Swami Sivananda

"America has the best doctors, the best nurses, the best medical technology, the best medical breakthrough medicines in the world. There is absolutely no reason we should not have in this country the best health care in the world." Bill Frist

CHAPTER SIX THE IMPORTANCE OF A SECOND OPINION

As I mentioned in the last chapter, in spite of the good news, I was still having feelings of uncertainty. I heard from a high school friend on Facebook. His son had an aortic aneurysm. He suggested that I contact his son's surgeon for a second opinion. I was very grateful for the recommendation and called her office and got an appointment made. She was also in the Charleston area, at Trident Medical Center.

I visited MUSC's records department and arranged for copies of my records to be sent to Dr. Karen Gersch. It was a rainy day going down to Charleston for the second opinion. In a way it was suitable; it was matching my mood. The dank gray overcast made for a dull and dreary day, a good day to be depressed. I'll admit now that trying to maintain a positive attitude every day was getting to be a strain. It was taking a great deal of effort to maintain a positive attitude, to keep my mind on a positive track. This visit was between my second and third visits to Doctor Katz at MUSC.

After signing in, I was taken to a waiting room. It couldn't have been more than five or ten minutes before Doctor Gersch entered. She had a lovely smile that brightened the day considerably. It turned out that she knows Doctor Katz. I explained that a friend had suggested I see her for a second opinion and she recognized his name.

We chatted for probably 45 minutes about my condition, the changes I was making in my life, etc. She affirmed that my starting to do some walking, as well as the dietary changes I had made, were all for the better; that they would help me in the long run.

I have to admit that, before I met Doctor Gersch, I was seriously considering asking her to refer me to a different doctor, or at least make a suggestion. But then she changed my mind on that. I was just concerned that it was taking too long at MUSC, that there were too many tests. She told me, without my asking, that, if she needed her Mitral Valve repaired, she would want Doctor Katz to do the job. She said that, short of going to the Cleveland Clinic or Harvard Medical School, I had the best surgeon for the job. Wow, you can't get a recommendation any better than that. While I had confidence in Doctor Katz before I went for the second opinion, the second opinion just helped increase my confidence level and reinforced my positive feelings that I was on the right course. She also took the time to explain the necessity for the tests in a way that I could understand. Doctor Katz had done that but his explanations just were not registering with me.

"The Christian's Bible is a drug store. Its contents remain the same, but the medical practice changes." Mark Twain

"Medical liability reform is not a Republican or Democrat issue or even a doctor versus lawyer issue. It is a patient issue." John Ensign

CHAPTER SEVEN POSITIVE MENTAL ATTITUDE

Let me reiterate that I am not a doctor, and I did not sleep at a Holiday Inn Express last night. I'm just going to relate what worked for me and why I believe that it worked. Your mileage may vary.

Your mind is a powerful tool when it comes to your body functioning. I remember being told years ago about a young man who had always been told by his mother that, if he was shot with a gun, he would die. He gets drafted into the army, sees action, receives a flesh wound in his bicep and promptly dies. There was no physical reason for him to die from the wound, but nonetheless, he did die. The only explanation available is that his mind had become so conditioned by his mother's "prophecy" that if he was shot, he would die, that the mind took over. He was shot; therefore, he must die.

I don't know if that story is true or not, but I do know about the "placebo effect," that the body can do things if the mind will let it.

I began a conscious effort to change my life. Mentally, I divided my life into "before surgery" and "after surgery" sections. I realized that I was being given a new chance at life and it was something that I did not need to waste. I began thinking about the changes I would make in my life.

The biggest change was in attitude. Looking back, I realize that I had been wondering a lot if things were worth it, if my life was amounting to anything, or if I was just going through time taking up space. I know that's a rather harsh assessment, but it is truly how I was feeling. I was seriously wondering what my purpose in life was. Post-surgery, I can tell you that I now know how Ebenezer Scrooge felt when he woke up after being visited by the three ghosts on Christmas Eve. While I'm still not absolutely positive about what my purpose in life is, I do feel that I'm meant to share my photography with people and that there are other things I'm meant to do. This book is, I believe, one of those things.

I had been waking up in the mornings with a "ho-hum, here's another day" attitude. I think that's a direct result of not knowing, or not believing, that there is a purpose to your life. I now start and end each day thanking God for the day and for the experiences I had. As I said, I think my purpose in life is to share the experience, the wonder, and beauty in the world around us. I now have a compass to guide me. As one of my business professors from college said, "If you don't have a plan, you'll hit it every time." While I may not have a formal plan, I do have a compass, a guide, to keep me heading in the right general direction.

Another "before surgery" change that I made was to start doing some walking. I walked around a local mall, averaging about ¼ mile a day. I did a slow pace as I did not want to aggravate the heart valve problem. The Mitral Valve (and the other heart valves) have "strings", like rubber bands, that pull the valve closed so there is no backflow of blood, no regurgitation. The "strings" had broken on my Mitral Valve, so it was not closing properly, forcing the heart to work harder to pump the same amount of blood and, at the same time, having to also fight the regurgitation. I did some reading and was able to conclude, based on what I had read, that the better condition you're in going into an operation, the better your recovery will be after surgery. Like I've said, I take whatever I see online with a huge grain of salt, but it did seem to be a logical conclusion. And neither doctor tried to discourage me from what I was doing. The only caveat I received was to listen to my body, in this particular instance, for shortness of breath, to make sure I was not overexerting myself.

Since the surgery, I'm up to walking about ½ mile a day, maybe even pushing a mile a day on the days when I'm back delivering food. I'm pacing myself, not pushing myself too hard, not getting myself exhausted. There have been a couple of times where I've had to take it easy for a day or two after delivering food because the delivery day was a bit long, or maybe a bit tiring. Still, I'm positive about my outlook on life, positive that I'm on the right course.

My good health is a gift, and it's a gift I hope I never fail to appreciate. I thank God each morning when I get up, and I thank Him each night when I go to bed for the beautiful day—even if that day has been filled with torrential downpours.

"No one should have to choose between medicine and other necessities. No one should have to use the emergency room every time a child gets sick. And no one should have to live in constant fear that a medical problem will become a financial crisis." Brad Henry

"You know what they call the fellow who finishes last in his medical school graduating class? They call him 'Doctor.'" Abe Lemons

"The good physician treats the disease; the great physician treats the patient who has the disease." William Osler

"The human body experiences a powerful gravitational pull in the direction of hope. That is why the patient's hopes are the physician's secret weapon. They are the hidden ingredients in any prescription." Norman Cousins

Like I've said, I dislike the word diet. It has too many negative connotations. I prefer "lifestyle changes." What you eat is an aspect of lifestyle, and it's important enough that I believe it is deserving of its own chapter.

You can go into any bookstore and you will find a plethora of diet books. There's Atkins, Keto, South Beach, and God knows how many others. I don't know for sure, but I assume that, to varying degrees, they all work. The trick is to find something that works for you, that you can live with. For me, it involved going to my mom's side of the family. Mom was first-generation Italian American, so the Mediterranean Diet was appealing to me. The Mediterranean Diet is more than just Italian food; Spain, France, Greece, and Northern Africa cuisines all enter into the mix. In my case I wasn't necessarily looking at specific cuisines, but rather a "diet philosophy;" in this case fresh foods: fruits, vegetables, meats, nuts, etc.

As I previously mentioned, the main protein in my diet is now chicken. It's fairly lean meat, and it absorbs marinades fairly well. This trait allows chicken to have a variety of flavors.

I try to stick to fresh fruits and vegetables. I do occasionally purchase canned fruits, generally something that is out of season. I try to find the fruit in a light syrup, to help in avoiding excess sugars. And let's face it, fruits do have a good bit of sugar in them. I avoid canned fruit cocktail, preferring to make fresh, generally with pineapple, grapes, blueberries, strawberries and maybe a few kiwifruits. It makes a nice refreshing change, especially in the summer.

A lot of diets say to avoid bread. Multigrain bread is really no different than plain white bread it just sounds healthier. Most refined grains lose up to 80% of their filling, heart-healthy fiber as well as up to half of their vitamins and minerals in the milling process. Whole wheat bread is healthier than white bread. For the same reason, whole grain bread is healthier than multigrain bread. Unless the label says that it is

100% whole wheat or 100% whole grain, it may still be primarily made from white flour. I tend to eat whole wheat pita bread which is made from yeast, sugar, flour, salt, and olive oil, it can be a good substitute for high-calorie traditional breads. I do sometimes have whole wheat "traditional" bread or whole wheat muffins.

For dairy, I usually have yogurt for breakfast. For the western pallet, it can take some getting used to. I tried several different brands and finally settled on Chobani "Flip". These are a flavored yogurt with a separate compartment that has some "crunchies" in it. You open it up, flip the "crunchies" in, and mix. These come in a nice assortment of flavors, including Key Lime Pie, Peanut Butter Crunch, and Boston Cream Pie. I tried fruit on the bottom yogurts but they didn't do it for me. I also, about once a month, will treat myself to some cheese.

If you're old enough, you might remember a time where no fat diets were paraded about as the cure-all. The problem is fats provide flavors you take those out and you need something else for flavor. Food producers settled on the other evil, salt. Because salt is bad for the heart, increasing blood pressure and water retention, it's something that I have cut back on considerably. As Julia Child was fond of saying, moderation. In fact, a lot of the foods that fit with the Mediterranean Diet off the shelf (bread, cheese, canned tuna, lightly salted nuts, etc.) have enough salt that you really don't need to worry about adding salt to your diet. When I go out to eat, I generally bring a grinder of either Italian herbs or Greek seasonings to add to my food. Either one adds flavor without adding more salt to your diet. And it's funny, once you start eliminating the salt, you realize that you don't miss it. You begin to really taste and enjoy the natural flavors of food, especially fresh fruits and vegetables.

One of the stickiest debate points in a heart-healthy diet is butter versus margarine. There was a time when butter was thought to not be heart healthy because of the high-fat content, although margarine has almost as much fat. Research has since found that saturated fat and dietary cholesterol found in butter tend to raise HDL cholesterol (the "good" one, which isn't linked with heart disease) and that they don't raise LDL cholesterol (the "bad" one). Instead, they actually improve

LDL, making it more benign and less harmful. This means that the saturated fat in butter does not increase the risk of heart disease, and many studies have confirmed this. Butter is an all-natural dairy product that's been around much longer than margarine. To make butter, cow's milk is shaken or agitated or churned until the fats separate from the liquid, which eventually results in butter. There are a few more steps involved, but that's basically how it's done. Some butter products have a few additives (such as salt or sometimes herbs) added to them.

	Butter (100 grams)	Margarine (100 grams)
Total fat	81 grams	71 grams
Saturated fat	51 grams	23 grams
Monounsaturated fat	21 grams	8 grams
Polyunsaturated fat	3 grams	37 grams

Margarine, on the other hand, is a man-made, highly processed product made from vegetable oil. Margarine was created in 1869 in France as a replacement for butter for soldiers and the lower classes, as butter was expensive. This means that margarine is similar in taste, appearance, and consistency to butter, but these similarities are achieved by adding a variety of artificial ingredients to margarine, including emulsifiers and artificial coloring. As well, margarine is put through a process of hydrogenation, which extends its shelf-life but also increases its trans-fat content.

Butter	Margarine
All-natural	Highly processed
Fewer additives; often has salt	Many additives, including coloring, emulsifiers, and other ingredients
High in saturated fat	High in trans fat
High in cholesterol	Low in cholesterol

While margarine used to be considered healthier, it's now believed that butter is the healthier choice. You will find health experts on both sides of the debate, but research has shown that saturated fat and dietary cholesterol aren't as bad as previously believed.

So, if you want to go with the healthiest choice, stick with butter. That said, eating too much butter still isn't good for you. In fact, a little bit of margarine is probably healthier than two whole sticks of butter, so remember to always eat in moderation and choose brands that are low in trans fats, as these will be healthier. If you don't like the taste of margarine at first, you can always try a few different brands.

Ultimately, with both butter and margarine, how healthy they are for you comes down to how much you eat. We need some fat in our diets for our bodies to function properly, but too much is bad for us. Butter is one great source of healthy fats. While there was a lot of paranoia and fear in the past about butter, spreading a little bit on your bread can be a healthy choice.

I have come down on the side of butter, although when I fry something if the recipe calls for 2 tablespoons of butter, I'll use between 1-1½ tablespoons of olive oil and ½-1 tablespoon of butter. Growing up in the South, I learned to like the flavor of butter when I was young and it's hard to totally eliminate the taste. And for baking, butter wins hands down.

The one thing I always do when I buy butter is to buy unsalted butter. There are three reasons for this. First, I don't need the extra salt. Second, you can't be sure how much salt will be in the butter. Third, in all likelihood, the recipe is going to call for some additional salt somewhere along the line. The main reason that butter wins is that it has a creamy texture that margarine just doesn't have. Butter imparts that texture to the food. And I hate to sound like a broken record but, as Julia Child said, moderation.

Now, with the help of the Mayo Clinic, I have compiled a list of foods to avoid.

First, anything with ingredients that you cannot pronounce. If you can't pronounce it, the odds are that it's artificial, and that goes against the philosophy of natural equals healthy.

Energy drinks seem to have generally negative health effects in addition to high amounts of caffeine and/or other stimulants which can be bad for heart health.

As previously mentioned, multigrain bread, whole grain is healthier.

Palm oils as they tend to have a negative environmental impact.

So-called "skinny" teas. These can act as laxatives to the body.

Anything called a "superfood." There is no such thing. There is no medical meaning or government definition of "superfood."

Gluten-free foods. If you need to avoid gluten, then, by all means, eat gluten-free. On the other hand, if you don't need to avoid gluten, then don't eat gluten-free foods.

Synthetic Growth Hormones, generally identified as BGH or BST. Anything that is artificial can't be all good for you.

As mentioned in the discussion on butter versus margarine, trans fats as they can cause health problems.

Excessive sugar. Sugar comes in many forms, Sucrose is table sugar but there are also other varieties, such as high fructose corn syrup, barley malt, maltodextrin, galactose, blackstrap molasses, agave nectar, honey, maple syrup, dextrose, and corn syrup. While many are natural, some are refined. Some are sugar alcohols which give the taste without being absorbed by the body. While that may sound like the best of both worlds, the downside is that they act as laxatives that can cause diarrhea. They are most often used in sugar-free foods.

While we're at sugar, "No sugar added" does not mean low sugar. It means exactly what it says, that no sugar has been added.

Sodium (salt) comes in many forms, monosodium glutamate (MSG), also known as Accent, sea salt, sodium nitrate, kosher salt, and disodium inosinate are just a few varieties of salt.

Any food that has "Natural" in the description. Natural has no nutritional meaning, there are no government regulations when it comes to using natural. There's no need to pay extra for natural.

Pasture-raised and free-range also have no meaning as there are no government regulations governing their usage.

Cholesterol free is a tricky item. All animals produce cholesterol, therefore the only way for something to be cholesterol-free is for it to have no animal products in it, i.e. a vegetable or fruit.

"I like the values associated with a medical family – common sense, being practical but also thoughtful." Alain de Botton

"I have enjoyed great satisfaction from my climbs of Everest and my trips to the poles. But there's no doubt that my most worthwhile things have been the building of schools and medical clinics." Edmund Hillary

"Three-quarters of the sicknesses of intelligent people come from their intelligence. They need at least a doctor who can understand this sickness." Marcel Proust

CHAPTER NINE EXERCISE

THIS IS IMPORTANT, SO I'M GOING TO SHOUT IT: NEVER, EVER, START AN EXERCISE PROGRAM WITHOUT CONSULTING WITH YOUR DOCTOR. I AM NOT A DOCTOR. WHAT I AM DISCUSSING IN THIS CHAPTER IS WHAT WORKED FOR ME.

Exercise is another key to good health. As we grow older, we tend to become sedentary; more sedate, more relaxed, especially when it comes to exercise and its benefits. It's something that goes hand in hand with getting older.

Exercise will improve your life, there's no doubt about that. The key is to gradually work into it, especially if you haven't regularly exercised in the past.

About five years ago, I started doing food delivery. I was walking probably about 1½ miles each day. The thing is, it was not constant walking, it was in short bursts. I honestly don't know how 1½ miles of cardio exercise in short bursts compares with 1½ miles of cardio exercise at one time. My gut feeling is that they are not the same; that the shorter bursts are not as effective as a longer continuous workout. At the same time, some exercise is better than none at all.

Unfortunately, I can't exercise just for the sake of exercising; there has to be a more tactile reason for me to exercise. I'm not wired to be a gym rat. Because of this, I've actually done an exercise throwback. Just about every child's first chance of freedom is a bicycle; it's a way to expand the limits of where you can go.

Back in the late 1990s, my dad had a heart attack and had to have a triple bypass. His father had died from a massive heart attack in the early 1960s at the age of 60. With that kind of family history, I knew that there was a pretty good chance that I would be having heart problems at some point in the future. I started to ride a bike for exercise. I eventually got up to riding about 25-30 miles a day and got to the point where, in 2000, I participated in Cycle North Carolina, a seven-day bike ride from Boone to Wilmington, covering between 400 and 500 miles. Unfortunately, I didn't keep up the bike riding, stopping about 10 years ago. I don't know if it helped me or not, or if it postponed my eventual Mitral Valve injury. Hopefully, I will be able to get back on the bike, maybe not with the intensity I had before, but maybe being able to ride three or four days a week, at an easy pace, just enough to keep the circulatory system primed and in good condition.

Returning to the present, before the surgery, I started walking about ¼ mile each day at the mall. Based on what I had read, the better your condition going into the hospital, the quicker your recovery from surgery would be. As I wanted to get the odds as much in my favor as possible, I figured that I would do all I could before the surgery to make my recovery as smooth as possible. During one of my visits to MUSC, I mentioned to Doctor Katz what I was doing. He asked if I was short of breath and I acknowledged that I was. His advice to me was to take things easy, listen to my body, and not to push things. I followed his advice to the letter.

I've said it before, shortness of breath is another thing that sneaks up on you. It doesn't hit you suddenly, it's a gradual change. It's insidious; it's so gradual that it seems like a natural part of living. I used my shortness of breath as a guide, as a way to make sure I wasn't overexerting myself during exercise. These gradual changes are often the hardest to notice because they are so gradual. Looking back, I can see clearly that another sign of shortness of breath was a consistent cough, especially when I tried to talk for extended periods of time.

"This is a really big space station. We do a lot of various kinds of work here, different kinds of science experiments; we have over 400 different experiments going on at any one time in different areas, from basic science research to medical technology, that hopefully will benefit more people on Earth." Scott Kelly

"Remember I'm a doctor's daughter. So obviously, I'm interested in all medical things." Nancy Reagan

"We should be concerned not only about the health of individual patients, but also the health of our entire society." Ben Carson, Secretary of Housing and Urban Development

"They certainly give very strange names to diseases." Plato

"I am dying from the treatment of too many physicians." Alexander the Great

CHAPTER TEN RETAINING FLUIDS

If you're retaining fluid, it's quite likely that your ankles are going to be one of the leading indicators. While other areas of your body will also retain fluids, the ankles are generally one of the most noticeable areas of fluid retention. Fluid can also be retained around your lungs and heart, and you'll feel that retention. Breathing will become harder, contributing to the shortness of breath. Again, before making any changes in your diet or exercise routines, consult with your doctor. The following is just general information.

Fluid retention, also called edema, is a pathological or non-pathological condition caused by an excessive accumulation of fluid in your tissues.

When it's pathological, it generally originates with circulatory problems, congestive heart failure, or problems with your kidneys or liver. When it is not, it is attributed to a simple dilation of your veins during times when temperatures are higher.

The consequences of fluid retention are:

Unexplained weight gain

Swelling in your legs and ankles

An increase in the size of your abdominal area or a decrease in your need to urinate.

Edema is mostly seen in older adults. However, it has also been diagnosed in adolescents. The condition is more common in women than men, especially for hormonal or dietary reasons. It also tends to appear during menopause, pregnancy or when a person has a sedentary lifestyle. However, fluid retention can be a sign that a person has another disorder, whether cardiac, renal, hepatic, or digestive.

How to tell if you have fluid retention:

1. Your lower extremities are swollen. Your lower extremities are the first part of your body to be affected by fluid retention,

so pay special attention to your legs and feet. At first, you'll feel tiredness and heaviness in your legs due to inadequate drainage.

2. Thicker ankles. Edema causes your ankles to look bigger than normal. From when you wake up until you go to bed, this part of the body increases in size as the day goes on.

3. Leg cramps. Going back to your legs, you will see swelling in them as well, though sometimes people don't notice it. One symptom that can reveal that you're retaining fluids is having frequent cramps in the area, along with weakness.

4. Bloating in your middle. Another area that's affected by the signs of fluid retention is in your belly. Some people think they're gaining weight when really, they are bloated. Some go on long, strict diets thinking that the increase in the size of their waist is fat when, in reality, it's a failure of your excretory system.

5. Swelling in your face. The swelling that comes from edema can also happen in your face. It is usually visible in your cheeks and eyelids, which will slightly increase in size. The excess of fluids makes your face appear rounder. Also, when you look at yourself in the mirror, you may notice that it's harder to see your eyes because your eyelids will have swollen.

If you think you may be retaining fluids, you can do the following:

Drink more water. It may seem counter-intuitive, but when your body retains fluids, it's because it is dehydrated. So, give it the water it needs. This way, it won't store it unnecessarily.

Go on a hypocaloric, low-sodium diet. When you're facing this problem, it's a good idea to reduce your consumption of refined flour and sugar, fat, and salt.

Exercise: It seems that this is a cure for all kinds of problems. Exercising will help you get rid of the extra fluids through sweat and urine, and also gets your circulation going. Your exercise routine should last at least 20 minutes a day.

Drink diuretic teas: Certain plants like dandelion, fennel, parsley, and green tea will help you go to the bathroom more regularly. You can also add vegetables like carrots and cucumbers to your diet, along with fruits like watermelon and melon.

Eat foods high in potassium: Corn, cauliflower, bananas, and asparagus can also help you out when you're retaining fluids due to their high potassium content.

Get rid of your dehydrating beverages: This is especially alcohol, the worst being beer and vodka, as well as coffee. As was explained above, when your body thinks it doesn't have enough water, it retains fluids.

Eat more protein: Chicken, red meat, fish, shellfish, and legumes are all good options. A lack of protein encourages fluid retention. I will have red meat occasionally, but it's not a major source of protein for me.

Don't wear tight clothing: It's unnecessarily uncomfortable and will make your body swell up a little more over the day.

Don't sit too much: If you're at your desk all day, get out of your seat for at least five minutes every hour. This way, your body won't enter into a sedentary state.

Stay away from too much heat: Stay away from environments that are too hot, since heat produces dehydration. When that happens, your body retains fluids.

"Deep-learning will transform every single industry. Healthcare and transportation will be transformed by deep-learning. I want to live in an AI(Artificial Intelligence)-powered society. When anyone goes to see a doctor, I want AI to help that doctor provide higher quality and lower

cost medical service. I want every five-year-old to have a personalized tutor." Andrew Ng

"Everybody should have access to medical care. And, you know, it shouldn't be a big deal." Paul Farmer

"When I told my doctor I couldn't afford an operation, he offered to touch up my X-rays." Henny Youngman

"Walking is man's best medicine." Hippocrates

CHAPTER ELEVEN THE POWER OF PRAYER

I want to start by saying that I have been thinking about whether or not to include this chapter since I began writing the book. I finally decided that I did need to include it because I believe that the power of prayer helped me with my journey through this almost year-long and life changing voyage. If nothing else, I know it helped me mentally.

One of the first things you do when diagnosed with a potentially life-threatening disease is to talk with family and friends about it, basically, let them know, let someone know. This is especially true if you have no immediate family. As things evolve along the journey, I found it useful, maybe even necessary, to be able to talk with friends about what I was experiencing. I'm sure that it helped me in coping with the situation. Having people to talk to who are not medical professionals, who can be a "safety net" if you will, can be very important.

Several of my friends are ministers of different faiths. I was put on prayer groups. As I said, I don't know if it made any physical difference. I know that as the visits to the doctor progressed, the surgical outlook improved from the most invasive (open heart) to the least invasive (robotic). Did the prayers make a difference? I don't know, and really, there is no way to tell for sure. The argument could be made that prayers did make a difference. The other side of the coin is that the increased number of tests were able to provide a better, more accurate, picture of what was happening and that knowledge changed the surgery prognosis.

At the same time, knowing that there were prayers did boost my spirits. Knowing that people cared about me enough to pray for me emotionally made a big difference in my life. It did lift my spirits. The light at the end of the tunnel was not another freight train.

In my mind, there is no doubt that knowing people were praying for me helped to keep me optimistic, that it helped with my positive mental attitude. Attitude is everything.

I'm not going to delve into religion here, just suffice to say that I do believe in God. As for the prayers, who is to say whether or not they helped or hurt me? I believe that they did help me, that they had a positive effect on the eventual outcome of this journey. Ask me to prove it? I can't. I have to accept it as a matter of faith.

"The mind controls so much of the body. We are much more than flesh and blood; we are complex systems. Patients do better when they have faith that they're going to do better. That's why I always tell my patients and their families not to neglect their prayers. There's nobody I don't say that to." Ben Carson

"A Harvard Medical School study has determined that rectal thermometers are still the best way to tell a baby's temperature. Plus, it really teaches the baby who's boss." Tina Fey

CHAPTER TWELVE SURGERY AND RECOVERY

It was right around Thanksgiving when I received a phone call from MUSC telling me that they had an opening for surgery on December 30th and asking me if I wanted it. There was no hesitation on my part, I jumped at the chance to get scheduled. The sooner I would have the surgery the sooner I could get back to living.

A dental exam was the last obstacle facing me. I opted to have the dental work done at MUSC mainly because of the HIPAA (Health Insurance Portability and Accountability Act), a 1996 Federal law that restricts access to individuals' private medical information. I figured having everything in the same hospital would make it easier for everyone; the dental school could simply add their clearance to my chart. There were a couple of glitches but I'm sure they weren't as bad as they could have been.

The week before surgery had yet another trip down to Charleston, this time for a final check and some lab work to make sure I was healthy enough for the surgery to take place. I was asked if I had a flu shot this year. I said that I hadn't and they went ahead and gave me one after assuring me that it would not affect my health or recovery. With everything looking good, I was given my final instructions. The biggies were to stop taking my medicines two days before surgery and nothing to eat after midnight the day of surgery. I would have to check-in at MUSC at 5:30 in the morning on Monday, December 30. I made a reservation at a Holiday Inn for the night before. They would let me leave my car at the hotel while I was in at MUSC and I would spend the night there before going home the day after I was released from the hospital. I did have the option of driving down to MUSC the morning of the surgery, but I opted, correctly I think, to go down the night before. I had to shower with a disinfectant soap the night before and the morning of surgery. I felt that I would probably be better off not doing the extra driving. I took a cab from the hotel to MUSC on the morning of the surgery, arriving there at 5:00 AM.

I got checked in and went up to the floor where the surgery would take place. They were remarkably efficient on the day of surgery. I was in a room by 5:45 and in a gown by 6:00 AM. I was partially shaved. Even though I was scheduled for robotic surgery and there was a less than 1% chance that they would have to do open heart surgery if, once they went in with the camera, they discovered an undetected problem, they wanted to be able to do the open-heart option without any delay. I do remember being asked about stents being put in, something along the lines of, "As long as we're in there, would you like us to check and see if stents are needed?" I agreed to that request, it simply made sense, check things out as long as they were in there.

By 6:30 AM, I was being wheeled into the operating room. I really have no recollection of what happened beyond this point. I was anesthetized and, after that, the rest of my chest and groin was shaved. For the surgery, I was put on a heart-lung machine and that connection was made at my groin. Surprisingly, the incision in that area was not painful.

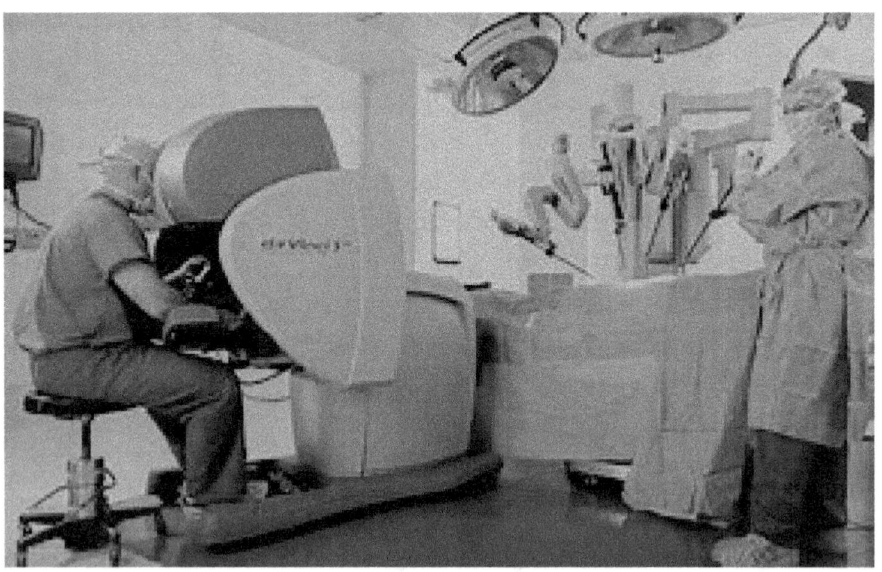

The DaVinci Robot—stock photo

Being anesthetized, I don't have firsthand knowledge of what occurred. I've read of people having out of body experiences during surgery. I'm not sure if I had an out of body experience or not. I remember seeing the DaVinci robot when I was brought into the operating room. I have a memory of Doctor Katz at the machine during the surgery, but it could be my mind playing tricks on me.

I don't know how long the surgery took. I do remember the nurse telling me before surgery that, once I was in the ICU for recovery, my vital signs would be taken every hour. Remarkably, I managed to sleep well, and soundly. I don't know if I woke up earlier, but I don't remember waking up until my vital signs were taken at about 3:30 AM on December 31st.

The robotic surgery was the least invasive surgery available. There were about five incisions along one of my ribs on the right side of my chest for the robot to have access to my chest and heart. My right lung was collapsed so that they could have access to my heart. An incision was made on the left side of my groin where I was connected to the heart-lung machine. Once I was connected to the heart-lung machine, my heart was stopped. A camera was inserted and the surgery was performed. The valve was repaired and a ring was inserted around the valve to help reinforce it. The incisions were sutured and a drain was installed for my chest. There was also a catheter to allow me to urinate. Surprisingly, it wasn't uncomfortable. Even when it was removed there was very little discomfort.

Doctor Katz came by shortly after I had breakfast on the 31st to see how I was doing. I told him that I felt fine and I wasn't in pain and he said the surgery went as planned and nothing unexpected showed up and no stents were needed. He said that, if my recovery continued has it had so far, that I could plan on being released from the hospital on Saturday (January 4, 2020). I remember thinking that would be great.

Shortly after Doctor Katz left, a nurse came by and asked if I would like to get out of the bed. I said that would like that very much and she helped me into a chair. I'm guessing I was in the chair for eight or nine hours. I remember that I had both lunch and dinner in the chair and went back to bed shortly after dinner.

At about 10 PM, I called for a nurse and asked her to bring two cups of ice. That was probably one of the stranger requests that she had heard from a patient, but she came in with the two cups. I told her that, in my suitcase, there was a brown bag and to please bring it to me. There was a momentary look on her face wondering if I had smuggled something illicit into the hospital. I had brought in a bottle of sparkling grape juice. I asked her to open it and join me in a toast to the new year. She laughed and readily agreed. After the toast, I told her that she could share the rest with the other nurses who were on duty that night. Before she left the room, she told me that I had one of the best attitudes that she had seen among patients. I smiled and told her that I could choose to be happy or sad and that my being sad wouldn't change the circumstances, so I might as well be happy.

New Year's Day was moving day in that I was moved from ICU into a private room. I also did three walks that day, one with a cardiac walker that I could rest my arms on padded surfaces, one with a regular walker, and the third walk I asked to not use a walker. I had to promise to stay close to the wall in case I started to feel like I was about to fall. I made that promise, and I was finally starting to feel "normal." On the last walk, without the walker, I thought of the scene from *Dr. Strangelove, or How I Learned to Stop Worrying and Love the Bomb*, where Dr. Strangelove rises out of the wheelchair and shouts, "Mein Fuhrer, I can walk!" and I started to laugh. The nurse, who was in her 20s, asked me what was so funny. I told her that I was just thinking of a scene from an old movie.

"I like old movies, which one?"

"Doctor Strangelove."

She started to laugh and whispered to me, "Don't you dare shout, 'Mein Fuhrer, I can walk!'"

At that point I started to laugh hard and had to lean against the wall to keep from falling over.

Again, I think that attitude means everything. I found myself channeling my dad's sense of humor during the stay. A nurse would come in and say. "You're looking good today," and I'd reply, "Thanks but I'm not good looking." Normally, I'm not one to do the snappy, wisecracking comebacks. At the same time, I think that my choice to be happy helped me remember some of my dad's sayings, and helped me to have a positive attitude. I spent most of the day sitting up in the chair, from just after breakfast until about 9 PM. I was also checked on by one of Doctor Katz's assistants.

There was one downside to being in a room. The catheter had been removed and both the bed and chair have weight sensors, in case you fall. This means that, if you need to use the bathroom, you need to call for a nurse. You can probably see where this is heading… I needed to go so I buzz for the nurse. I get an answer and tell her what I needed. She said would be there in just a couple of minutes. They had a problem arise, and over ten minutes pass. Finally, I couldn't wait any longer so I was faced with one of two options. I could either go in the bed and they would have to clean the bed and me, or else I could get out of bed and walk to the bathroom, and set off the alarm indicating that I wasn't in the bed. I chose the second option. Of course, they come running in while I'm in there going. I simply explained that I couldn't wait any longer and I figured my getting out of bed and setting off the alarm would be the least objectionable, and certainly the least embarrassing, option.

Hospital food tends to be the butt of numerous jokes. There may have been a time when hospital food did live down to that reputation. I have to say though that, at least at MUSC, the food was good; not gourmet by any means, but it was enjoyable and had some flavor to it. I found the pot roast to be one of the better offerings on the menu, so much so that I had it twice while I was there.

Thursday, January 2nd ended up being a day of surprises. I woke up and had fruit for breakfast. I had an early morning visit from Doctor

Katz and he told me that I could go home that day. I told him that I couldn't. He looked at me quizzically and I said, "You gave me so much Lasix today that I'm peeing about every 15 or 20 minutes. I won't be able to make it from Mount Pleasant to McClellanville (the next town with public restrooms) without having to stop on the side of the road to go. It did get a chuckle from him. Fortunately, I had my backup plan, the hotel where I had left my car, a Holiday Inn.

The hospital concierge called and was able to get me a room, and the hotel sent their courtesy van. It's nice when hotels and hospitals have a good working relationship, it helps make things go smoother for the patient—and the patient's family. By noon I was checked in at the hotel. I went to the dining room for a light lunch and I returned that night with a friend for dinner. I have to give kudos to the Holiday Inn at the Ashley River. They were one of the nicest hotels I've ever been to, in terms of the staff being willing to work with guests, especially when they are facing surgery of some type. While I'm talking about things working together, I have to compliment MUSC. Everyone there was exceptional. It seemed like everyone was on the same page; there were not any failures to communicate. There was one concern that MUSC had, and that was they had called in my prescriptions to my pharmacy in Myrtle Beach. Fortunately, I had all my prescriptions for the day so the only potential problem was if I experienced any pain.

Pain is a sensation that is "relative," there is no precise measure. The doctor may ask how much it hurts on a scale of 1-10, but there is still no precise way to measure the level of pain, it's not like blood pressure; a five for one person might be an eight for someone else. I told the hospital that it would not be a problem. I had not had any pain medication, other than acetaminophen since the morning I woke up from the surgery. They insisted on giving me pain medication that day. That night I said let me try without it and I slept fine. I was confident that I could sleep without it, and that proved correct. After not using the pain medication for over two months, I finally took it to the local police department for disposal.

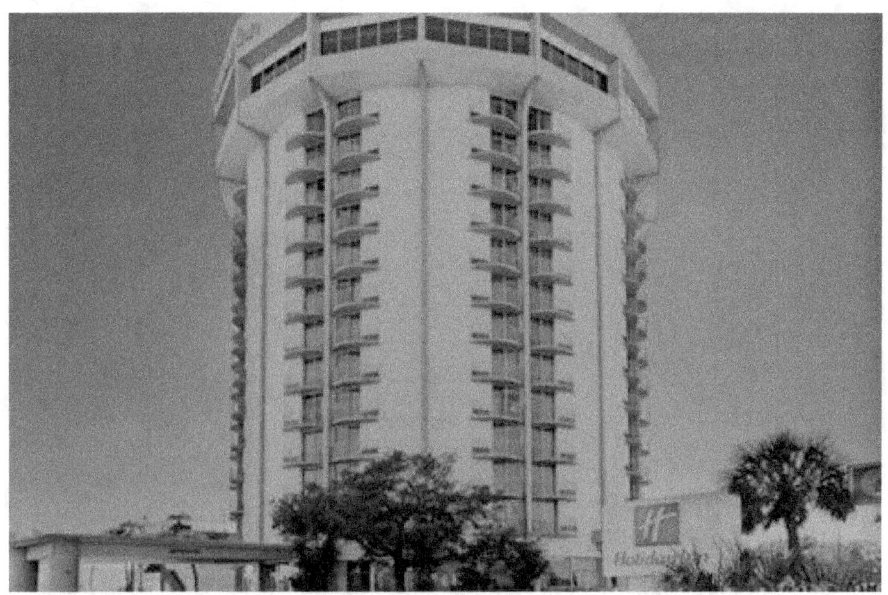

Holiday Inn Ashley River

Another reason for choosing this Holiday Inn was that their restaurant is open for breakfast, lunch, and dinner. The restaurant's placement, on the roof, was an added bonus as it afforded absolutely spectacular views of Charleston, the oldest city in South Carolina. This hotel is also round, so I was able to make several laps on my floor during the day, inside, at a nice comfortable temperature.

January 3rd, I checked out of the hotel and pointed the hood of my car north towards Myrtle Beach. It was a new year and a new life. Over the past four days, my life had dramatically changed for the better.

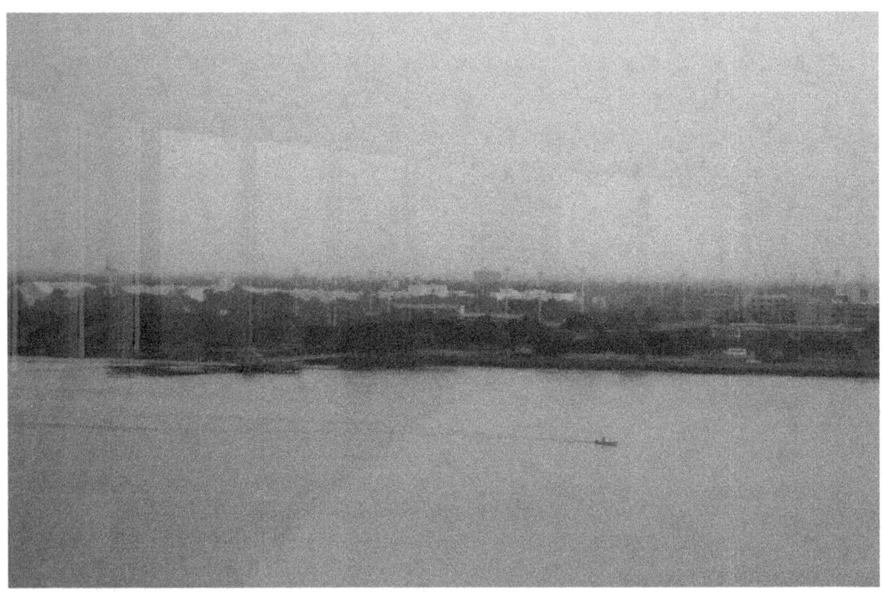

A view from the restaurant at the Holiday Inn Ashely River. The Ashley River is in the foreground, the Citadel, the military college of South Carolina is on the left and in the far back are cranes from the Wando Terminal of the State Port Authority.

"When medical students focus on helping others, they're able to weather the slings and arrows of long hours and devastating health outcomes: they know their colleagues and patients are depending on them." Adam Grant

"In the real world, 90% of the money spent on medical research is focused on conditions that are responsible for just 10% of the deaths and disability caused by diseases globally." Peter Singer

CHAPTER THIRTEEN THE FIRST MONTH

I took my time driving home. There was no rush. In fact, I now realize that many of the deadlines we place on ourselves are artificial. I've undergone a lot of changes. One of the first is that I've come to value time, not that I didn't value it before. Maybe the correct term is that I now have a better appreciation of time, an appreciation of that, once it's gone, you can't get it back.

When I checked out of MUSC, there were no firm directions given to me as to what or what not to do. Rather, it was more common-sense guidance. Be active but listen to your body. Don't cause excess strain on yourself. When I was discharged, I could only lift my right arm about shoulder high before the pain from the incisions would set in. Each day I would raise my right arm, three or four times a day, and very slowly I noticed my arm was going higher and higher.

I made a point of getting dressed and going out each day. It's far too easy to become homebound. I went to the mall each day, walked about ¼ mile, and spent a lot of time listening to my body. I used a cane just to help steady myself. Even though I hadn't been off my feet that long, I still felt a little wobbly when I was on my feet.

Each day I felt myself getting stronger, able to take a few more steps than the day before. It was a new aspect of the journey. I was in the hospital for only four days, yet I felt that I was physically almost starting over from scratch.

I had thoughts of the progress I was making, wondering if it was real or a figment of my imagination. At the end of the first week, I had to make another trip down to MUSC. I met with a nurse and told her how I was doing. She was pleased with the progress I was making. We talked for a while. She gave me some additional guidance, mainly to make sure that I was paying attention to my body. She said that they were concerned that I not try to do too much too soon.

It was a wonderful visit. It confirmed what I had been thinking and that I was on the right track. I could slowly increase the amount of my exercise as long as I paid attention to the signals from my body.

I gradually increased my walking distance each day by a few steps. I was feeling better each day. By two weeks out of the hospital, I wasn't needing the cane every day. There were times when I felt I needed it, and would carry it with me, but I began to listen a little closer to my body. I could soon differentiate between "needing" the cane versus "wanting" the cane. I still keep it in the car, just in case I feel the need for it when I'm making a food delivery, and there are rare occasions when I do need it.

About three weeks after discharge I was up to walking about ½ mile each day. I've been maintaining that distance since then and until I meet with my local cardiologist.

On January 30th, I had a final trip down to MUSC to meet with Doctor Katz. It was a month after the surgery. I was feeling great. Before I was diagnosed with this problem, I was thinking that I was just experiencing what 62 years old felt like. Now I feel like I'm ten years younger. There are still rare occasions when I feel short of breath, but those are few and far between and generally occur after I've done some exercise. It's all a matter of learning to listen to my body.

That visit included a final meeting with Doctor Katz. I'm a semi-professional photographer and I had one of my photographs printed in color 20 inches by 30 inches on aluminum. I call the picture *"Sea Oats at Sunrise."* At the end of the visit with Doctor Katz, he said that I was cleared and he didn't want to see me anymore. I then gave him the picture and told him that it symbolized what he had given me. I had a new life, almost like a new day, and that I was looking forward to exploring the gift that he had given me. It turned out that he also does photography as a hobby and he was very appreciative of the image.

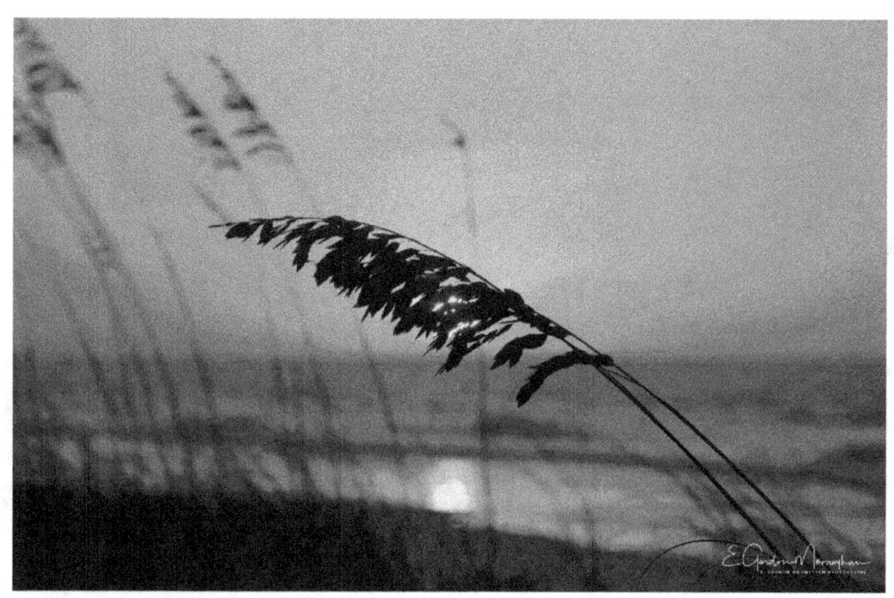

Sea Oats at Sunrise, copyright 2020, E. Gordon Mooneyhan

"In the 20th century, we had a century where at the beginning of the century, most of the world was agricultural and industry was very primitive. At the end of that century, we had men in orbit, we had been to the moon, we had people with cell phones and color televisions and the Internet and amazing medical technology of all kinds." David Gerrold

"Medical attention is medical attention, whether it's for your elbow or for your teeth or for your brain. And it's important." Jon Hamm

CHAPTER FOURTEEN CARDIAC REHAB AND BEYOND

On February 26, 2020, I had a visit with my local cardiologist. It went well. He confirmed that there were no blockages and that I was indeed, able to return to work. I was a bit taken aback when he asked me if I wanted to enroll in cardiac rehab. I asked why, since there were no problems and he said that it would help me learn how to take better care of my heart, what I could and couldn't do in the way of exercise and, in general, help improve my overall health. That was almost a no brainer and I agreed that it would indeed be helpful to me.

Cardiac rehabilitation, also called cardiac rehab, is a customized outpatient program of exercise and education. Cardiac rehabilitation is designed to help you improve your health and help you recover from a heart attack, other forms of heart disease or surgery to treat heart disease.

Cardiac rehabilitation often involves exercise training, emotional support, and education about lifestyle changes to reduce your heart disease risk, such as eating a heart-healthy diet, keeping a healthy weight and quitting smoking.

The goals of cardiac rehabilitation include establishing an individualized plan to help you regain strength, preventing your condition from worsening, reducing your risk of future heart problems, and improving your health and quality of life.

Research has found that cardiac rehabilitation programs can reduce your risk of death from heart disease and reduce your risk of future heart problems. The American Heart Association and American College of Cardiology recommend cardiac rehabilitation programs.

Cardiac rehabilitation is an option for people with many forms of heart disease. In particular, you may benefit from cardiac rehabilitation if your medical history includes:

- Heart attack

- Coronary artery disease

- Heart failure

- Peripheral artery disease

- Chest pain (angina)

- Cardiomyopathy

- Certain congenital heart diseases

- Coronary artery bypass surgery

- Angioplasty and stents

- Heart or lung transplant

- Heart valve repair or replacement

- Pulmonary hypertension

Don't let your age hold you back from joining a cardiac rehabilitation program. People of all ages can benefit from cardiac rehabilitation. Well, I have two of the items on the list, heart failure, and heart valve repair, and I'm pushing senior citizen status. This was another case of not knowing, of not keeping up with medical advancements. I was thinking that cardiac rehab was only for people who had heart attacks or bypass surgery.

Generally, you will go through a series of stages:

Medical evaluation. Your health care team will generally perform an initial evaluation to check your physical abilities, medical limitations and other conditions you may have. Ongoing evaluations can help your health care team keep track of your progress over time.

During your evaluation, your health care team may look at your risk factors for heart complications, particularly during exercise. This can help your team tailor a cardiac rehabilitation program to meet your individual needs, and the team can make sure it's safe and effective for you.

Physical activity. Cardiac rehabilitation can improve your cardiovascular fitness through physical activity. Your health care team will likely suggest low impact activities that have a lower risk of injuries, such as walking, cycling, rowing, jogging and other activities. You'll usually exercise at least three times a week. Your health care team will likely teach you proper exercise techniques, such as warming up and cooling down.

You may also do muscle-strengthening exercises, such as lifting weights or other resistance training exercises, two or three times a week to increase your muscular fitness.

Don't worry if you've never exercised before. Your health care team can make sure the program moves at a comfortable pace and is safe for you.

Lifestyle education. You'll usually receive support and education on making healthy lifestyle changes, such as eating a heart-healthy diet, exercising regularly, maintaining a healthy weight and quitting smoking.

Your health care team may give you guidance about managing conditions such as high blood pressure, diabetes and high cholesterol.

You'll likely have opportunities to ask questions about such issues as sexual activity. Don't be too embarrassed to ask questions. It's highly unlikely that you will ask something that hasn't been asked before. You'll also need to continue taking any medications you've been prescribed by your doctor.

Support. Adjusting to a serious health problem often takes time. You may feel depressed or anxious, lose touch with your social support system, or have to stop working for several weeks.

If you get depressed, don't ignore it. Depression can make your cardiac rehab program more difficult, and it can impact your relationships and other areas of your life and health.

Counseling can help you learn healthy ways to cope with depression and other feelings. Your doctor may also suggest medications such as antidepressants. Vocational or occupational therapy can teach you new skills to help you return to work.

Although it may be difficult to start a cardiac rehabilitation program when you're not feeling well, you can benefit in the long run. Cardiac rehabilitation can guide you through fear and anxiety as you return to an active lifestyle with more motivation and energy to do the things you enjoy.

Cardiac rehabilitation can help you rebuild your life, both physically and emotionally. As you get stronger and learn how to manage your condition, you'll likely return to a normal routine, along with your new diet and exercise habits.

It's important to know that your chances of having a successful cardiac rehabilitation program rest largely with you. The more dedicated you are to following your program's recommendations, the better you'll do.

After your cardiac rehabilitation program ends, you'll generally need to continue the diet, exercise and other healthy lifestyle habits you learned for the rest of your life to maintain heart-health benefits. The goal is that at the end of the program you're confident to exercise on your own and you're empowered to maintain a healthier lifestyle.

Cardiac rehabilitation is a long-term maintenance program, and you'll generally need to continue the habits and follow the skills you learned in the program for the rest of your life. After about three months, you likely will have developed your own exercise routine at home or at a local gym.

You may also continue to exercise at a cardiac rehab center, a fitness center or a club. You may also exercise with friends or family. You may remain under medical supervision during this time, particularly if you have special health concerns.

Education about nutrition, lifestyle and healthy weight may continue, as well as counseling. To get the most benefits from cardiac rehabilitation, make sure your exercise and lifestyle practices become routine. In cardiac rehab you will, over the course of the program, be given pamphlets with information to help with your recovery.

Over the long term, you may:

- Gain strength

- Learn heart-healthy behaviors, such as regular exercise and a heart-healthy diet

- Cut bad habits, such as smoking

- Manage your weight

- Find ways to manage stress

- Learn how to cope with heart disease

- Decrease your risk of coronary artery disease and other heart conditions

One of the most valuable benefits of cardiac rehabilitation is often an improvement in your overall quality of life. If you stick with your cardiac rehab program, you may come out of the program feeling even better than before you had a heart condition or had heart surgery.

Everything had been going smoothly but then the Covid-19 outbreak hit and hospitals were closed for elective procedures. My cardiac rehab ended up getting postponed for almost three months. That was really the only hitch in the entire process.

I tried getting back on my bicycle but I quickly discovered that I could not stand the heat anymore. Before surgery, I had been told that I might experience some changes, that people react differently to surgery. In talking with the nurses in rehab I found out that it was possible, if not probable, that the change in my ability to tolerate hot weather was likely due to either one of my medications or, more likely, a combination of the medications that I was taking, along with some particular aspect of my metabolism.

The actual rehab was a completely different process. The course of the exercise you undergo is a function of the medicines you take as well as the surgery you've had. In my case, I was told that my "ideal" heart rate while exercising is 10-20 beats above my resting heart rate. I asked this after my first week of rehab because I found I was getting tired at work.

I talked about this with the nurses. There's more t delivering pizza than just hopping in your car and walking to the guest's front door: there's prep work that's involved, taking care of sorting the truck first thing in the morning, etc. There's a lot of work that isn't thought of when you say your job is delivering pizza. We determined that my physical activity at work was at a higher level than they thought it would be, so my exercise regimen was adjusted. It did seem to make a difference.

To help pace myself at work I bought a Pulse-Oximeter. If you've ever been in the hospital, you know that little gizmo that the nurse will slip. on the end of your finger? That's a Pulse-Oximeter. It does two things, first it measures your pulse and second, it measures the amount of Oxygen in your blood. I bought mine online for less than $30. I brought it to the hospital for one of my rehab sessions and we compared its readings with the $500 unit in cardiac rehab. They were identical. Now I have a way to track my pulse rate while I'm exercising.

Cardiac rehab was, for me, a 12-week class and I decided to put off writing this chapter until I had completed the course. It started out for me as an ordeal because, as I said earlier, I couldn't exercise for the sake of exercising. But something would happen along the way.

Endorphins.

Endorphins are chemicals released by your body that reduce the perception of pain in your body. It's a high that some people have likened to morphine. Generally, they will give you a mood and energy boost for two or three hours and a mild buzz that can last for up to 24-hours. What happened was I wanted to break the tedium or monotony of the exercises I was doing, so I started doing intervals where I would warm up at an easy pace, then push myself hard for a couple of minutes, return to a comfortable pace for a few minutes, and repeat. I was releasing endorphins, like I did when I was riding my bike. I was giving myself a natural high. In the process, quite by accident, I discovered the secret to enable me to enjoy exercising in a gym.

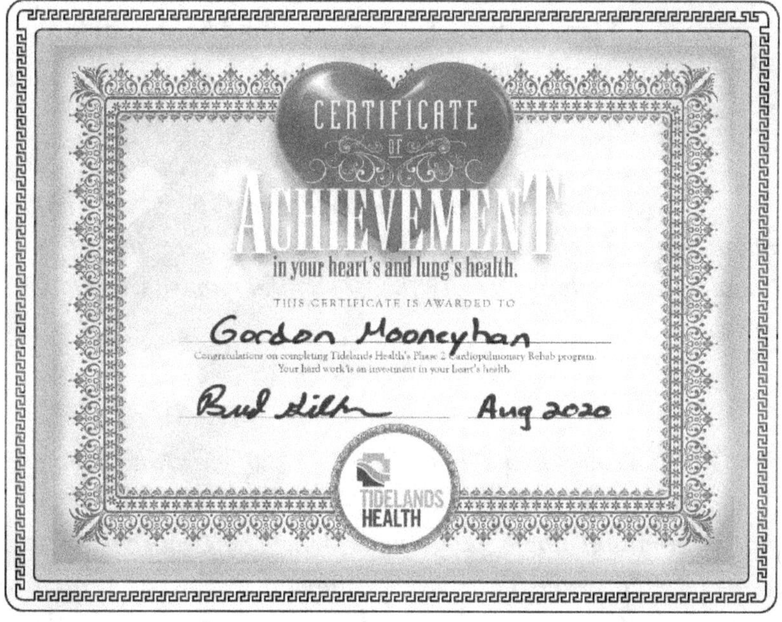

My certificate showing that I successfully completed cardiac rehab.

Now that I've finished cardiac rehab, I want (and need) to continue the exercise program that I've started. If you have family, there's your support group. They can help keep you motivated. Since I live alone and with no family in the immediate area, I rely on friends and co-workers to keep me motivated. So far, it's been working. My routine goes something like this. On my days off from work, I'll do about an hour of cardio at Planet Fitness. On the days I work, I'll go after work and do 30-45 minutes of strength training. Generally, I make Saturday and Sunday my rest days. I'm managing to get somewhere between 3½ and 4¼ hours of exercise each week, in addition to the exercise I'm getting making deliveries. When I left cardiac rehab, they suggested that I try for about 2½ hours each week. I'm passing that goal by at least an hour each week.

I realize that it's not essential to exercise in a gym; I could just as easily engage in walking. The thing is that the nurses at cardiac rehab said to keep my heart rate when I exercise and 10-20 beats per minute (BPM) above my resting heart rate, or between 90-100 BPM. The cardio equipment at Planet Fitness has sensors you can hold onto that will let the machine display your heart rate.

"My most important projects have been the building and maintaining of schools and medical clinics for my dear friends in the Himalaya and helping restore their beautiful monasteries, too." Edmund Hillary

"It's crazy to me that in this world of electronic medical records Walmart has so much information about how we shop, but no one has that information about our health. Why can't my doctor say, 'Wow, Anne, based on your lifestyle and behavior, you're five years from being diabetic.' But I can go to Target and they know exactly what I'm going to buy." Anne Wojcicki

CHAPTER FIFTEEN HINDSIGHT IS 20/20

This chapter is a look back at events leading up to the surgery, some of which haven't been covered in other chapters mainly because they don't fit anywhere else. Another reason for this chapter is that heart disease is the leading cause of death. If some of the signs that I've experienced can warn someone else that they might be having a problem and cause them to seek treatment, then I will have done some good writing this book.

As I've said, these are events that, for the most part, don't appear suddenly. The changes are slow to occur and, being slow changes, they are hard to notice, and they really don't become noticeable until looking in hindsight.

Upon reflection, I think the first signs that something was wrong had probably occurred about a year or so earlier. I noticed that, when I was at work preparing food, that I would occasionally be out of breath. It wasn't anything consistent, but just occasionally. Oddly enough, I didn't notice any problems when I was delivering food. I can't explain why this was, but I can speculate. I assume it was because I was doing enough driving, sitting and resting, that I was able to catch my breath so that the shortness of breath wasn't as noticeable, compared to when I was preparing food, which was an hour or so of continuous work.

The shortness of breath gradually got worse over time. I found that I would need to take a minute or two to catch my breath while prepping the food. Again, as I've said before, it's insidious. It creeps up on you, like a thief in the night. It was so gradual, that I quite honestly believed that I was just experiencing what 62 was supposed to feel like.

I also noticed that my ankles were starting to swell a bit, nothing that I thought was alarming, and the swelling would go down overnight. I didn't put two and two together; I didn't realize that I was retaining fluid. That's one of the signs of heart failure, but I wasn't aware of that at the time.

As time went by, I noticed that I was having a harder time breathing. I was having to pace my talking if I tried talking too much, or too fast, I would have coughing fits. It was the shortness of breath manifesting itself in another way; yet another sign of congestive heart failure.

As I said, the situation kept getting worse and, upon reflection, the decline in my health was probably increasing at a faster pace. By the end of 2018, I would have to take a couple of five-minute breaks to catch my breath while prepping food in the morning. Again, in hindsight, this should have been perfectly clear to me and alarm bells should have been going off. But in real life, the change was so gradual that it either wasn't that noticeable or else it was easy to dismiss as part of growing older.

Since early 2019 was more of the same, let's fast forward to March 9, 2019. It was a Saturday, a pleasant spring day, shirtsleeve weather. It was nice to be delivering food with the car windows open, inhaling the fresh sea breeze. I had a big pizza delivery at the end of the day to the Ripken Baseball Experience in Myrtle Beach—28 pizzas. I guess about halfway through going back and forth to my car, I really lost my breath. I started huffing and puffing like a steam engine. Somehow, I managed to finish delivering the order. I got back to my car, turned on the air conditioning, and sat there for about ten minutes, catching my breath. I finally felt well enough to drive back to the store. I had the next two days off and I spent them relaxing, catching up on light chores that I needed to get done around the house. I think it's important to note that I did not feel any pain when this happened. At the same time, with hindsight being 20/20, I would be willing to bet that this was when the strings that controlled my Mitral Valve broke. Proof? I don't have any physical proof. The only proof I have is how I felt after that event. I thought I had been out of breath before, that was nothing compared to how I was feeling now. To use a southern expression, I felt like I'd been hit upside my head with a 2x4. This was the wake-up call that I so desperately needed. I made up my mind that, if I wasn't feeling better in two weeks, I would get my tush to the doctor.

Well, life got in the way. I was so busy with work that I lost track of time and it was almost a month later before I got to the doctor and received the diagnosis of Congestive Heart Failure. That was the real wake-up call, especially when I found out that Congestive Heart Failure was no longer a death sentence.

"Let's all be humbled about the evidence behind medical advice but also respect the challenges to providing accessible lifestyle guidance." Dean Ornish

"It's a medical fact that children can have a better chance in life with better looks, better health and more vigor if the teeth, nose, throat and mouth are taken proper care of at the crucial time of childhood." George Eastman

CHAPTER SIXTEEN WHAT THE FUTURE HOLDS

Since the surgery, I realize that I've been given a second chance, a new outlook on life. I've always had a belief in God, although I don't attend church on a regular basis. I believe that God used this opportunity to get my attention, to whack me upside my head with the proverbial 2x4. I feel that we all have a purpose in life, but I wasn't sure what mine was. I think I know now, and this book is one aspect of why I was allowed to survive; to share my experience with others, to alert them to health hazards and take proactive action.

I also have a deep admiration for the natural beauty that is all around us, whether it's a beautiful sunny day, the angry side of nature in a violent storm, the quiet beauty of a landscape, or the beauty in a piece of architecture. Both North and South Carolina have places of immense natural beauty. I think one of my missions is to share that beauty with others. I'm sure that if I get off track too much that God will give me a gentle nudge to get me focused again. I know He can put the 2x4 away.

"And now you know the rest of the story." Paul Harvey

ABOUT THE AUTHOR

E. Gordon Mooneyhan is a freelance writer and photographer in Myrtle Beach, SC. A native of Connecticut, his father moved the family back to South Carolina when Gordon was in the fourth grade. They then moved to Myrtle Beach when Gordon was a freshman in high school.

Gordon has photographs that are in the private collections of many artists, as well in the collection of the Mystic Seaport Museum. His photography can be viewed at his website **http://gordon-mooneyhan.pixels.com** .

Gordon is also an amateur chef and has had a lifelong interest in railroads. He combined his interests and has published three books on Amazon of railroad dining car recipes. One from the Southern Railway, the Atlantic Coast Line Railroad, and the Seaboard Air Line Railroad.

Gordon is also an amateur radio operator and Public Information Officer for the Grand Strand Amateur Radio Club. In 2018, he was the recipient of the Philip McGan Award presented by the American Radio Relay League, the national association for amateur radio, in recognition for his outstanding efforts in promoting amateur radio.

www.ingramcontent.com/pod-product-compliance
Lightning Source LLC
Chambersburg PA
CBHW050654250726
48662CB00002B/669